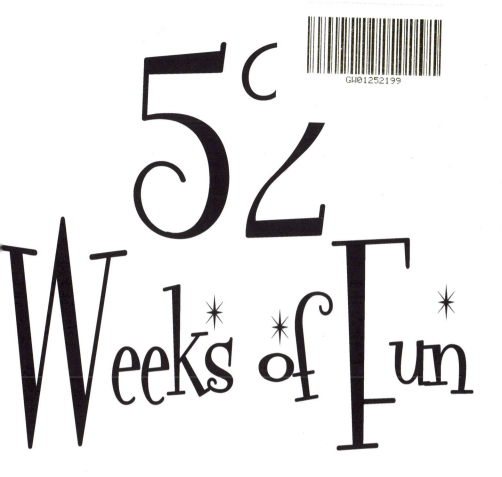

Have a Girls' Night In Every Week of the Year

Laura Jonsson
with Sarah Anthony & Lisa Walsh
Illustrations by Andrew Twite

First published in 2012 by
Laura Jonsson
Mona Vale, NSW 2103
AUSTRALIA
laurajonsson@hotmail.com

Copyright © 2012 by Laura Jonsson

All rights reserved. No part of this publication may be reproduced, stored in a retrieval system, or transmitted by any means, without the prior permission in writing of the publisher.

Library of Congress Cataloging-in-Publication Data
is available from the publisher.

ISBN: 978-0-9886708-0-8

www.52weeksofFun.com

This book is available at quantity discounts for bulk purchases.
For information, please email laurajonsson@hotmail.com.

Contents

Acknowledgements		7
Introduction		9
1.	Miss Mix-A-Lot	11
2.	Personal Styling Session	13
3.	Sips & Strokes	15
4.	Favorite Flicks Fest	17
5.	Silly Olympics	19
6.	Roll Out the Red Carpet	21
7.	Karaoke Queens	23
8.	Mani, Pedi & Martini Party	25
9.	Around the World	27
10.	Naughty or Nice Night	29
11.	Saturday Night Fever	31
12.	Celebrity Heads	33
13.	Breast Friends	35
14.	Sushi and Sake Soiree	37
15.	Clothes Swap	39

Contents

16.	Spring Fling	41
17.	Viva Las Vegas	43
18.	Train Your Brains	45
19.	Hawaiian Luau	47
20.	Down the Rabbit Hole	49
21.	Trivial Pursuits	51
22.	Uncork a Book	53
23.	Moroccan Fantasy	55
24.	Wii Love to Compete	57
25.	Green-thumb Gathering	59
26.	Sizzlin' Summer Soiree	61
27.	Wild West Hoedown	63
28.	Promise You Won't Be Board Game Night	65
29.	Progressive Dinner	67
30.	Hardback, paperback, do you want this book back?	69
31.	Mexican Fiesta	71
32.	Ice Cream Sundays	73
33.	Be Dazzling	75
34.	Croquet, anyone?	77
35.	Dollars & Sense Dinner	79

Contents

36.	Howdy, neighborini!	81
37.	Star Gazing	83
38.	WhoDunIt? Dinner	85
39.	Oktoberfest	87
40.	Fondue You Want to Come Over for Dinner?	89
41.	Hey baby, what's your sign?	91
42.	Stitch N' Bitch	93
43.	Bond Girls	95
44.	Side-dishes and Leftovers for Dinner	97
45.	Aroma-rama	99
46.	Card It Up Catch-up	101
47.	Girls Just Wanna Have Fun	103
48.	Cookie Exchange	105
49.	Perfect Match	107
50.	Best Dressed	109
51.	Reach for the Stars	111
52.	Wine Club	113
Drinks Recipes		115
Food Recipes		119
Suggested Song Lists		123

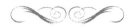

"I get by with a little
help from my friends."

~ John Lennon

Acknowledgements

There are several people who made this book possible. Lisa Walsh came up with the idea with me almost three years ago and my sister, Sarah Anthony, encouraged me continuously since then to complete it. They are two of my closest girlfriends and I am so lucky to have them both in my life!

Lisa's brother, Lee Walsh, had the idea for the title for *52 Weeks of Fun*, which allowed me to complete this book in half the time. My brother, Andrew Twite, did an outstanding job with the illustrations and I greatly appreciate his contribution. It is thanks to the graphic design mastery of Tina Henry, Ian's cousin, that the cover design was finally completed. And while I'm on family, my parents, Brenda and Tony Twite, for their love and support and Mimska, the world's-best-mother-in-law. Also, my amazing Grandma, Marjorie (aka Pat or Midge) Hamilton - I hope that when I am 92 I am in as good physical and mental shape and still have my childhood girlfriends like she does!

In my lifetime I am extremely fortunate to have some of the best girlfriends a woman could ever want. A special shout out to Megan, Samantha, HB, Malee, Nookie, Christian, Christi, Meredith, Kris, the old crew of girls from V3 (Kathi, Kerstin, Kimberley, Julie) the fabulous girls I worked with at Sirona (Sylvie, Deanna, Jen, Marcella, Melissa, Trish, Eva), Law, Susan, Katie, Mariel, Jules, all the girl's in Alex Mac's wine club, the fabulous group of girls I work with at Investec (El, Lyndall, Laura T, Tracy, Robs and Cindy), Jill and Sarah. While I'm not in touch with all of these women now, I had some great girl-time with all of them and want them to know that they are special to me and how much I appreciate their friendship.

Finally, and most importantly, my husband, Ian. He is the most supportive, loving partner and the best father for our boys. I love you Punkle!!

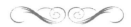

"I have chosen to be happy because it is good for my health."

~ Voltaire

Introduction

Women need their friends like plants need the sun. While men tend to go into isolation when under stress, new research studies show that when women are stressed they seek out other women to bond with. Their friendships improve their health by lowering blood pressure, cholesterol and heart rate. How often have you heard a girlfriend say, "I need a girl's night"? Well, it's not just idle chatter, or a flippant disregard for the men in our lives – it's a scientifically proven fact– we NEED to have fun with our girlfriends!

But sometimes sitting around and chatting or bellying up to a bar just isn't enough. And sometimes after a stressful week at work or with the kids, our brains just can't seem to come up with any fun ideas.

This book has 52 great ways for you and your friends to entertain each other and since there is one for every week, you can have fun all year! Whether you are a babe-on-a-budget or a lady-living-in-luxury, there are suggestions to cater for everyone. The weeks are not in a set order, so choose your nights in accordance with your mood and the season.

There are links to instructional websites and there are sections in the back of the book with music suggestions, drink and food recipes. Look for these icons to find more info:

- Additional web resources - bottom of the page
- Drink recipes - page 115
- Food recipes - page 119
- Suggested song lists - page 123

While drinking is mentioned on several of the nights, it is certainly not a requirement to have a fun time. But if you do want to enjoy a few adult beverages, make sure to be responsible and have a plan for everyone to get home safely!

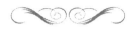

Guide to Mixers

Crisp
Bitters
Cranberry
Soda water
Tonic

Dry
Bitters
Champagne
Soda water
Tonic

Fizzy
Champagne
Cola
Soda water
Lemon-lime soda
Tonic

Fruity
Cranberry juice
Grape juice
Orange juice
Pineapple juice
Tropical fruit juice

Sour
Fresh squeezed lime juice
Fresh squeezed lemon juice

Sweet
Chocolate syrup
Cola
Cream of coconut
Orange juice
Lemon-lime soda
Pineapple juice
Simple syrup

Fresh Ingredients and Garnishes

Berries
Celery stalks
Cocktail onions
Limes (slice, twist or wedge)
Maraschino cherries
Oranges
Pineapple (slice or wedge)
Sugar (granulated or powdered)
Carrot sticks
Cinnamon
Lemon (slice, twist or wedge)
Mint (sprigs or leaves)
Olives
Pepper
Salt (Kosher salt)

Miss Mix-A-Lot

Get a bev-ucation in Mixology with your best mates.

Making a good drink is not just a skill - it is an art form that now has a proper name, Mixology. You can find Mixology classes in all of the trendiest cities and it is very easy to host one of these events at your own home; all you have to do is ask each guest to bring a specific spirit, mixer and garnish. If you don't have a variety of glassware, ask guests to bring what you need from their homes. For a list of must have spirits, mixers, garnishes and glassware visit the BarBack website and follow the links to "Stocking a Home Bar" and "Necessary Equipment" on the left-hand navigation bar.

The Miss Mix-A-Lot Mixology event is about two hours long and starts with a little bev-ucation. You will need an intoxicologist (instructor), who could be a drink-savvy friend or invite a bartender that you know is up to speed on the latest cocktails.* The intoxicologist will educate you on the history of a few types of liquor (Gin, Vodka, Rum and Tequila) and then teach you about different kinds of drinks (sweet, sour, dry). While they are presenting, the intoxicologist will make drinks for everyone to sample and get you ready for the really fun bit…

…the Miss Mix-A-Lot competition! Split guests into teams of two and have each team design their own cocktails. They will need to decide the ingredients, presentation (glass and garnish) and give their special drink a brand (name and character). Have each team present their cocktails to the other teams, who will sample them and then judge on taste, presentation and name. The team with the most points will be crowned Miss Mix-A-Lot!

A small tip…we've found the fruity, sweet drinks are always a crowd pleaser and give you better odds of winning!

*Of course, if you don't drink alcohol you can always make virgin versions.

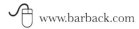 www.barback.com

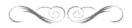

"Fashions fade, style is eternal."

~ Yves Saint-Laurent

Personal Styling Session

*Models and celebrities have personal stylists
and you can, too!*

Tired of wondering: "Does my butt look big in this?" We all enjoy wearing clothes that flatter our shape, but it can be hard to know what suits us. Hire a professional stylist to come over and give you some great advice or pick up a book and do it yourself.

A good stylist will know how to dress all body shapes and have an understanding of color and how it interacts with a person's complexion. They will also be able to create styles that match your individual personalities and ages.

Your personal stylist, or a good personal styling book, will give you tips on:

- what clothes to buy that suit your body shape
- how to dress appropriately for your age while still looking young and stylish
- what to wear for specific occasions
- what goes with what in your wardrobe
- how to spend less and yet have more to wear
- what to buy and where to buy it
- topping up wardrobes for new season looks with simple accessories and fashion

Once you have found your colors you could do makeup as well, or book it in for another night!

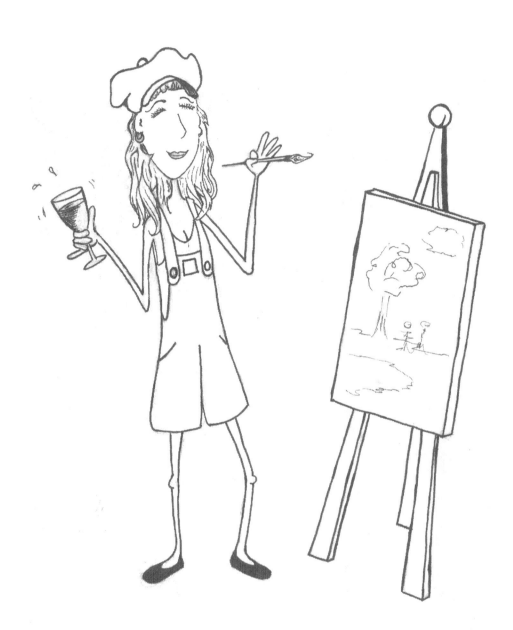

Sips & Strokes

Get your creative juices flowing while sipping on your favorite beverages.

Remember the early days when no one forced you to color between the lines or questioned the accuracy of your drawings? This night is not about being "an artist". It is about having a little fun playing with your friends. Even guests whose artistic skills don't go beyond drawing stick figures will enjoy an evening of loosening their creative inhibitions.

Set up easels with lots of paper and have a selection of art materials, such as crayons, watercolors, markers and colored chalk. Encourage your guests' creativity by letting them pick their paint (or other medium) and their poison (everyone should bring a bottle of their favorite wine). Ask friends who are particularly artistic to give brief tutorials to those who are interested in learning.

If you need help coming up with a subject to paint, ask everyone to bring something from home for some inspiration. To make it a bit more interesting, try life drawing and hire a local model for you to doodle.

Create a display area to showcase everyone's work at the end of the party by stringing a clothesline across the room and have guests clip on their creations. Take pictures of each work of art and upload them to a digital album so your guests have copies of everyone's artwork and can get inspiration for future projects.

Nobody's judging, but after a few drinks they all look like masterpieces!

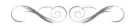

"No form of art goes beyond ordinary consciousness as film does, straight to our emotions, deep into the twilight of the soul."

~ Ingrid Bergman

Favorite Flicks Fest

*No matter what genre you and the girls are into,
a movie marathon is always a hit.*

Chick flicks are one of the best categories for a girls' night as there are so many good ones and yet so few that you can convince male partners to watch with you. There's nothing like watching a good tearjerker with good friends, just make sure you have plenty of tissues on hand!

Musicals and classic films are a close second to chick flicks in the "I can't get my partner to watch these movies with me" competition. You could all sing-along with the Sound of Music or drool over Paul Newman and Robert Redford in Butch Cassidy and the Sundance Kid.

Comedies are a great pick if you've been in a bit of a slump or have been super-stressed. Check out a documentary or two if you'd like to learn about something new or need a little inspiration.

There's no better way to watch a scary movie than in the dark with your friends. Horror flicks can range from slightly comical to sleep-with-the-light-on-for-three-days-after-scary, and it helps to have someone you can scream with, without being told you're too girly!

These are just a few suggestions and if you don't feel like a whole night of one genre you could start with a horror, laugh off the fear with a comedy and end the evening with an inspiring love story. Or, have everyone bring their own favorite movie and choose three at random.

As long as you have plenty of popcorn, treats 🍴, and good company, whatever you decide to watch will be a hit!

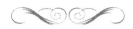

Silly Olympics Tally Board

	Team 1	Team 2	Team 3
Sack race			
Tricycle race			
Egg & spoon race			
Water balloon toss			
Jump rope contest			
TOTAL			

First place = 3 points
Second place = 2 points
Third place = 1 point

Silly Olympics

A more fun and less expensive way to stay youthful.

Remember how much fun the sports carnivals were in elementary school? Well, what better way to stay young at heart than by spending an evening competing against your friends in the Silly Olympics? You don't need to be athletes to participate in these games – just be ready to ditch your dignity and play to win!

Divide everyone up into teams and keep it fair by pulling names out of a hat. Before the night, create a scoreboard with a bit of poster board and list all of the events down the side and then add the team names up top on the night.

If you are creative, you can invent your own silly games that combine a mixture of skill, balance and concentration. If you need some inspiration, there are over 60 games to choose from on the NBC game show "Minute to Win It" website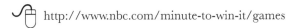 and in addition to a video tutorial, each of the games has instructions and a list of the items required for the game.

If you have outdoor space and the weather is nice, then you can compete in sack races, tug-of-war and borrow little tricycles to race around an obstacle course.

Choose ten to fifteen games and for each one have all teams choose one member to compete.

If you serve pizza and beer you can use the pizza boxes and beer bottles or cans for many of your events. To make it a bit more interesting, get creative with drinking penalties for fouls on certain games!

As always, prizes for the winning team are great, but bragging rights are usually enough of a reward.

http://www.nbc.com/minute-to-win-it/games

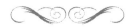

"We want to thank all of you for watching us congratulate ourselves tonight."

~ Warren Beatty

Roll Out the Red Carpet

Everyone will be a celebrity at your own award show night.

The Academy Awards ceremony is one of the most prominent and oldest award ceremonies in the world. Most of us will never get an invitation to the Oscars, but you can host your own Oscars party that is sure to get great reviews!

Line your entrance with a bit of red carpet and create a mini-theatre in your TV room. Ask each guest to dress as one of the characters from the nominated films (don't forget the animated and foreign films, too) or wear their most red-carpet-worthy dress.

Have a little competition to see who has the best eye for talent and can pick who 'the Oscar goes to…' in each category. Make it interesting by creating a pool and having cash prizes for winners.

The show goes on for hours, so be sure to have plenty of food and drinks on-hand. Finger foods and a selection of hot and cold canapés 🍴 can be put out on a table for guests to enjoy throughout the evening.

If you really want to extend the party, once the nominees are announced you can get together once a week in the month leading up to the show to watch one of the movies up for the "Best Picture" award.

There are enough award shows that, if you wanted to, you could be Rolling Out the Red Carpet every weekend for months on end and do them all!

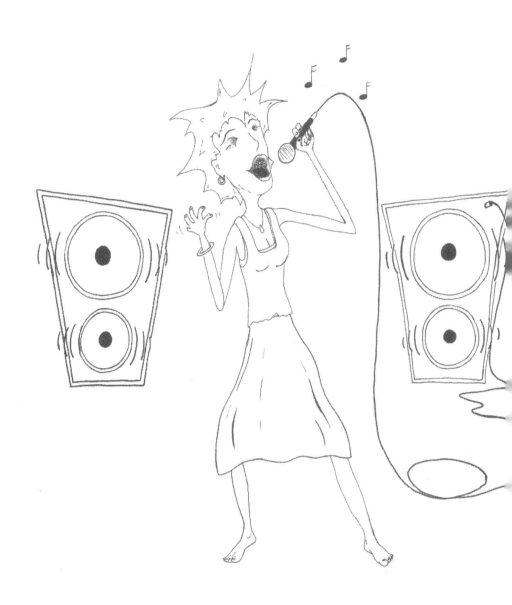

Karaoke Queens

Unleash your inner-diva and impress your friends with your singing skills.

Whether you are tone-deaf or a serious contender for the next season of Idol, this night can be fun for everyone. There are several karaoke systems available nowadays from SingStar® to cheap machines that you can buy at local toy stores and plug straight into your TV; if you or any of your friends don't already own one, it is definitely worth the investment! If you don't want to spend the money then check if your cable TV provider has a karaoke station you can turn to and just fashion your own microphone (hairbrushes or wooden spoons will suffice). ♪

For your shy friends, you might need to have a few shots of liquid-courage on hand to help coax them onto the stage, or just remind them that we're all friends here and it doesn't matter if they can't carry a tune. But if they just really don't want to sing, there's always room for back-up dancers! Or bring along a few triangles or tambourines – whatever it takes to get everyone involved.

Many of the karaoke systems will give you a score for your performance, however, don't worry if you don't score well; I am positive that I sing better than my tone-deaf husband, but I add my own flare to songs with unscripted oohs and ahs so he often scores higher.

Competition or not, sharing your musical talents with friends is always fun!

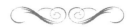

"I believe in manicures. I believe in overdressing. I believe in primping at leisure and wearing lipstick. I believe in pink. I believe happy girls are the prettiest girls. I believe that tomorrow is another day, and... I believe in miracles."

~ Audrey Hepburn

Mani, Pedi & Martini Party

*You'll have a fun night nailed with your
home salon and martini bar.*

You and/or at least one of your friends is bound to have a foot spa buried away in a cupboard somewhere and this is a great time to get it out and prove to partners or roommates that it is not just wasting space! If you don't have a foot spa, a few cheap Tupperware tubs will do the trick.

If you're on a tight budget, ask everyone to bring bath salts, lotions, and nail-maintenance kits. If money is no object, splash out for latest spa kits at your favorite boutique or salon. You'll need two clean towels for everyone, so if you don't have enough ask guests bring their own. Also, make sure you have the latest trashy mags to catch up on all the gossip!

Ask everyone to bring a few of their favorite nail polish colors; since a nail salon in your own home is free, it is a great time to try a new, crazy color. If any of you have an artistic flare, then get glitzed-up with a little nail art.

French Martinis are a perfect match for French Manicures and are easy to make.

This night is great a day or two before a big event, especially if it's the season for open-toed shoes…just make sure you let the polish dry properly before you enjoy too many martinis!

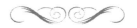

Popular Ethnic Cuisines

	Appetizer	**Main**	**Dessert**
Brazilian	Acarajé (fried balls of shrimp, black-eyed peas, and onions)	Feijoada (black bean stew with smoked meats that takes a full day to prepare)	Passion Fruit Mousse
Chinese	Egg Rolls	Sweet and Sour Chicken	Almond Cookies
Greek	Olive Tapenade	Baked Lamb with Potatoes	Baklava
Indian	Vegetable Samosas	Butter Chicken	Pistachio and Saffron Rice Pudding
Italian	Tomato and Basil Bruschetta	Lasagna	Tiramisù
Mexican	Guacamole with Tortillas	Fish Tacos	Tres Leches Cake
Thai	Chicken Satay Sticks	Pad Thai	Mango Sticky Rice Pudding

Around the World

*Experience other countries' cultures
without leaving your 'burb.*

We can't all afford to jet set to exotic locations to learn more about different countries, but with a bit of creativity you can experience many different cultures at home in one evening. Pick a few different countries for every course and explore their food, drinks, traditions, and culture in general.

Ask your guests to bring an ethnic dish from their own culture or their favorite international cuisine, as well as a representative song. ♫ With approximately 195 countries in the world you have plenty of options. Make sure to discuss your guests' choices beforehand so that you can coordinate to be sure that each course represents a different culture or region, and that your dishes will compliment each other.

If you've got the time and skill, print up menus with all of your dishes and an interesting fact about the country that makes the dish. Decorate with flags and maps and trinkets from the countries you will be exploring (think German beer steins, Mexican piñatas, stamped Moroccan lanterns).

Regardless of your destinations, everyone is bound to have a good time when you think global and party local!

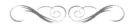

*"When I'm good,
I'm very good,
but when I'm bad,
I'm better."*

~ Mae West

Naughty or Nice Night

Lingerie and adult toy party

No matter how prudish or wild your group of gal pals is, this night can be as tame or raunchy as you desire!

You'll have to arrange a party consultant from an adult toy company who will actually do most of the party planning for you; you'll find all you have to do is decide who to invite and what to eat. The consultant will bring along their latest and most popular products and can even provide the entertainment if you are interested in having a few party games.

You will have to provide, or have each guest bring, some finger foods and appetizers. For a bit of fun make phallic cupcakes! Make sure that there is enough wine or spirits to get everyone in the mood.

Once everyone has had a bite to eat and a little drinky-poo to loosen up, you all sit around in a circle and the consultant will show you their lingerie, novelties and adult toys. You pass everything around the circle for all to get a closer look, and even have a little taste of the body sauces or sprinkle the body dust with feather ticklers.

After everyone has had a chance to see what is on offer, the consultant will go into a separate room and guests can go and privately try on any lingerie and discreetly order whatever tickles their fancy!

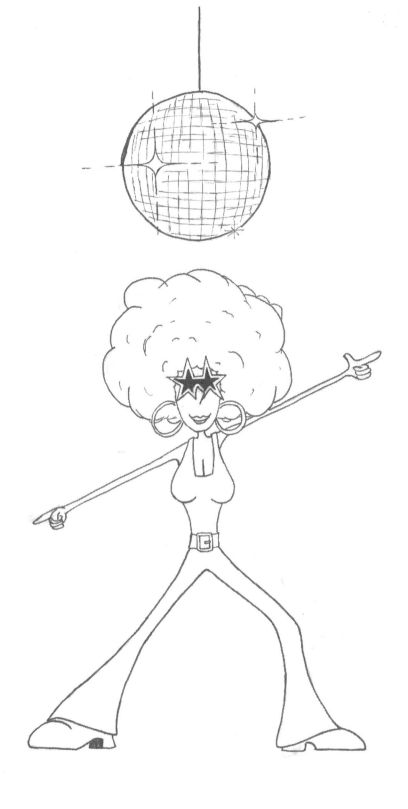

Saturday Night Fever

70's Disco dance party

Put on a bell-bottom jump suit and ask all the foxy ladies to do the Hustle to your place for a 70's disco dance party!

Decorate in earth tones like brown, orange and yellow and a little bright green and blue. Hang beaded curtains and get out a few lava lamps and the mood will be set. A rotating mirror ball is a must and make sure there is plenty of space for a dance floor where you can show off your groovy moves to The Village People, ABBA and the Bee Gees.

Fancy dress is a great way to make sure your party is far out, so ask your guests to come as their favorite 70's icon. Here are three ideas:

- Suzanne Somers (as Chrissy from Three's company) – tracksuit jacket, short shorts, sneakers with knee-high athletic socks and a side ponytail
- Farrah Fawcett – button down shirt with butterfly collar, high-waist denim flares, feathered hair
- Diane Keaton (as Annie Hall) – baggy pants, vest, necktie and fedora

The food of the 70's was about as appetizing as the décor. Start with devilled eggs, green and black olives and Clams Casino and then move quickly into main dishes of meatballs on a toothpick with jam sauce, pita pocket sandwiches and hamburger helper. Side dishes like mac 'n' cheese and broccoli casserole were popular in the 70's. A Jello mould will be the icing on the cake for dessert. Wash all of that down with some Harvey Wallbangers and Daiquiris and you'll be ready to hit the dance floor.

Can you dig it?

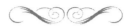

"A celebrity is any well-known TV or movie star who looks like he spends more than two hours working on his hair."

~ Steve Martin

Celebrity Heads

"Am I male?", "Am I short?", "Have I had an affair with Hugh Grant?"

Have you ever wanted to be a celebrity? Well this is game is your chance...the only thing is you won't know which celebrity you are!

A fun and easy-to-understand game, all you need to do is write down the names of well-known celebrities (dead or alive, sports, TV, movie, etc.) on post-it notes or index cards and put them into a hat. Everyone picks a name out of the hat and without looking at it sticks it on her forehead. The goal is to be the first to guess your celebrity name.

Mingle for a bit and then sit in a circle. One person starts, asking the person to their left a yes or no question about their celebrity. If the answer is a yes, the player asks the next person in the circle a question. If the answer is no, the player's turn is over and play rotates to the left. Keep going around the circle until someone correctly guesses their celebrity name and wins the game.

You could also include 10 blank name cards to allow your guests to create additional celebrity names or develop their own unique names, for example:
- friends, coworkers and family members
- type of sports
- household items

You can play this game for hours and it is guaranteed that a good laugh will be had by all.

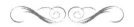

Breast self-exam: What to look for

1. Lumps or hard knots - may or may not be painful to touch
2. Swelling, warmth, redness or darkening of the breast
3. Change in shape or size (increase or decrease) of the breast
4. Unusual thick areas inside the breast or underarm area
5. Any changes in the skin of the breast or nipple - wrinkling, dimpling or puckering
6. Itchy, scaly red rash or sore on the nipple
7. Pulling in (inverting) of your nipple
8. Nipple discharge (green and sticky or bloody)

Breast Friends

*Raise awareness and spirits with a
night in for breast cancer.*

Breast cancer is the most common cancer found in females and almost everyone knows someone who has been affected by this disease.

To help raise awareness of breast cancer and money for your local cancer charity, host a pink party where everyone wears pink. Invite guests to give what they would normally spend on a night out as a donation to a breast cancer foundation.

One in nine women will be diagnosed with breast cancer and therefore early detection is vital, so as part of the evening you could also demonstrate self-examination basics. The easiest way to do this is by watching a short instructional video on YouTube. Make a list of symptoms to look for (see opposite page) with a reminder that if you notice any to see your doctor immediately to have them checked.

To add to the pink theme, decorate with pink balloons and table linens and make up a batch of pink cupcakes, which you can serve with pink fairy floss (cotton candy) and pink lemonade. Fondue using pink marshmallows and chocolate is also a yummy treat.

http://www.nationalbreastcancer.org/
http://www.nbcf.org.au/

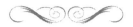

When the character of a man is not clear to you, look at his friends.

~ Japanese Proverb

Sushi and Sake Soiree

Enjoy the Far East without the long flight and crowds.

Put on your kimonos and take off your shoes for an authentic Japanese evening. Decorate with paper globe lanterns and have low tables with cushions where you will eat.

You can either order sushi and sashimi platters or if you are keen make your own hand-rolled sushi. All you have to do is provide various fillings, which could include sliced cucumber, carrot, avocado, tuna, salmon, or any other sashimi. Arrange these ingredients on a plate and have a large bowl with plenty of cooked sushi rice and a plate of nori seaweed. Give each guest a plate and small dishes for soy sauce, wasabi and pickled ginger. Guests can use a spatula to spread the rice onto the seaweed, choose their own ingredients and then roll up their creations.

For the seafood avoiders, you can offer Chicken Katsu or a beef noodle dish on the menu. Green tea is also a must and will add to the ambiance if you can serve it in a Japanese tea set.

A few fun activities could be karaoke, which is very popular in Japan, Mahjong or learn to make your own origami cranes, which are meant to be good luck.

You can serve hot sake and make sure you have plenty of Japanese beer on-hand (Kirin Ichiban and Asahi are good choices). If you are up for it, sake bombs are always fun!

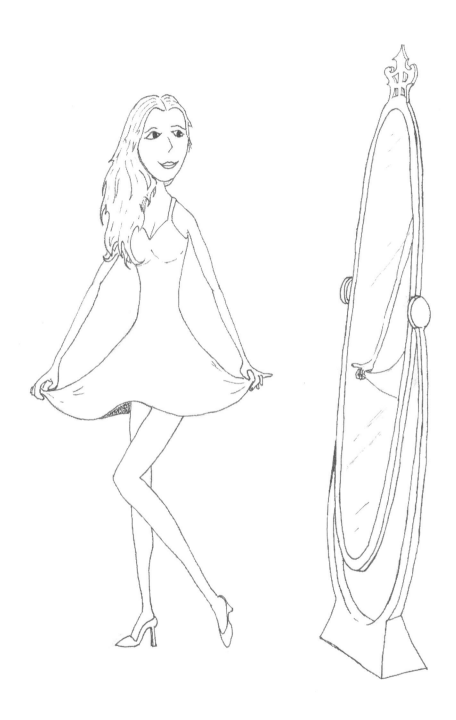

Clothes Swap

Enhance your wardrobe with free new clothes by hosting a fashion exchange.

Experiencing an all-too-familiar fashion crisis and yet have a closet full of perfectly decent clothes? Then why not improve your wardrobe by swapping instead of shopping? Many of your friends are in the same situation and you can all save money and enjoy some fabulous new outfits and accessories with a clothes swap.

Ask all of your guests to bring at least three items (clothing, accessories, purses) they no longer use and would like to trade. Bring items that are likely to be valued by your friends, who will not want your old pilled, stained or stinky tracksuits, leggings, undergarments, etc. All garments should be in good condition, clean and folded or pressed.

As your guests arrive, give them one token for each item and then arrange clothing by size and style and put like accessories together, like a boutique. Setting up can take up to 30 minutes, so have cocktails and canapés ready for everyone to enjoy and make sure you enlist the help of at least one guest to help you get set-up.

Once everything is neatly arranged you can open your boutique and let the swapping begin! To keep it fair, swap one-for-one and keep track by collecting a token for each item. Everyone leaves with something new!

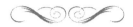

"Spring is nature's way of saying, 'Let's party!'"

~ Robin Williams

Spring Fling

*A garden party brunch to celebrate
the end of winter months.*

After a long, cold winter a great way to come out of hibernation is at a garden party with your friends. If you don't have a garden, you can easily use a decent-sized balcony, rooftop terrace or turn your indoor space into a garden with potted plants, flowers and floral decorations.

A fun activity to get you into the spring season is to invite a floral expert or a green-thumbed friend for a basic flower-arranging lesson. Ask guests to bring a variety of flowers and their favorite vases and learn different arranging styles and tips on helping flowers look better and last longer. Everyone will leave with a new skill and a beautiful arrangement to enjoy at home!

Serve fresh, seasonal food and don't forget to share any food or herbs you've grown in your gardens. A selection of teas and sandwiches are always a winner and if you're in the mood for an adult beverage then mix-up a pitcher of refreshing Mint Julep.

All of your guests are sure to have a bloomin' good time!

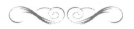

Blackjack terms

Term	Meaning
bust	having a total over 21, resulting in an automatic loss
double down	placing an additional bet equal to original bet and subsequently drawing one and only one additional card (this move may only be used on the first two cards)
first base	the betting spot located to the dealer's left, which is first to receive cards and first to act
hard hand	hand that doesn't contain an ace that is valued as 11
hit	take another card from the dealer
holecard	second card dealt to the dealer that is dealt face down and not revealed to players until after they have acted upon their hands
insurance	if dealer shows an ace, players can place a side bet of half the value of the original bet (if the dealer has blackjack - the player gets his wager back plus the original bet, if the dealer doesn't have blackjack - the player loses his wager)
push	a tie; player and dealer hands have same total
soft hand	a hand that contains an ace valued as 11, as opposed to 1
stand	to stop asking for more cards (aka stand pat, stick, stay)
stiff	any hard hand where the possibility to exceed 21 exists by drawing an additional card namely 12,13,14,15 or 16
surrender	abandon your hand, while recovering half your initial bet
third base	the betting spot located on the dealer's right, which is last to act
upcard	the card that the dealer is showing

Viva Las Vegas

Casino party

If a trip to Vegas isn't on the cards, you can still get a little Vegas action by turning your home into a casino. Invoke the glitz and glamour of Vegas with sparkling lights and a motif of spades diamonds, hearts and clovers in red and black - perfect casino colors. Sparkly silver and gold ornaments and decorations will add pizzazz to the event.

Ask guests to come in cocktail dresses and get cheap costume armbands and green plastic dealer visors. Put on music by the Rat Pack or Elvis Presley to add to the Vegas ambiance. ♫

Black jack, craps, and Texas Hold'em poker are all fun table games that are easy to set-up. If you've got the funds, home poker kits with cards, chips and a nice playing surface are easy to find on the Internet. You can also make a nice table cover with a bit of green felt from the fabric store. Make sure you have enough chips for everyone; at least 35 per person, but preferably 50-100. Ask your guests to bring some extra chips of their own if you don't have enough. If you're playing Texas Hold'em, make sure you have a special chip for the button.

Finally, don't forget the food and cocktails and serve on plates, cups and napkins decorated with dice, cards or dollar signs. You want finger foods that are easy to eat so that your guests can focus on the games. The real casinos know that the best way to get your money is to keep the drinks flowing and dirty martinis, scotch on the rocks or vodka-lime-and-soda are perfect cocktails.

Odds are everyone will leave feeling like a winner!

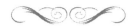

"The nice thing about doing a crossword puzzle is, you know there is a solution."

~ Stephen Sondheim

Train Your Brains

*Clear the cobwebs with a clever little contest
to test your craniums.*

If you and the gals haven't been behaving like a bunch of brainiacs recently and you're starting to feel a little mentally sluggish, plan a night of brain-stimulating activities to sharpen your cerebral skills. Mental exercise is just as important as physical exercise, especially if you've been killing off a fair few brain cells with fun nights out.

Activities that will help stimulate your brain can include crosswords, Sudoku, and memory games. Have all of your guests bring enough copies of their choice of game for everyone, or just ask them all to bring their laptops and play online. Make it a bit more interesting with a little competition by comparing your results.

Serve foods that will increase your brainpower like salmon sandwiches and blueberries with yogurt. Research has proven that the scent of peppermint helps you focus and boosts performance, so brew up a batch of peppermint tea.

It goes without saying, but too much alcohol makes you sloppy, not sharp. However, a drink or two can increase arousal signals, so a couple of martinis made with the uber-popular Super-food Acai may make you all as sharp as tacks!

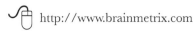 http://www.brainmetrix.com

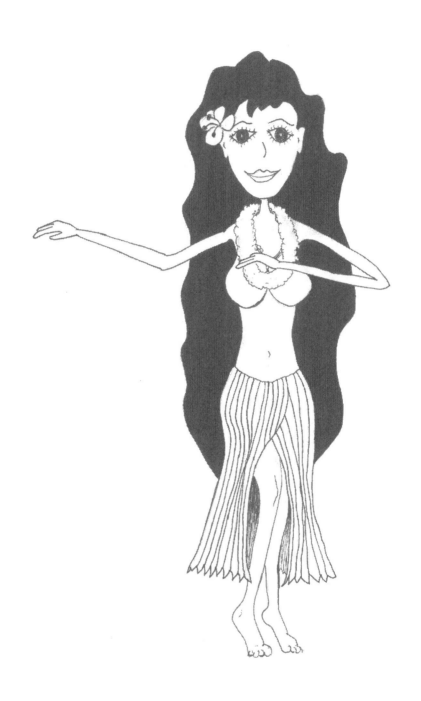

Hawaiian Luau

Journey to your own Land of Aloha to enjoy an evening of tropical paradise.

Best in summer months at a backyard, courtyard or rooftop terrace, just turn up the Island music and you will be transported to your tropical Hawaiian Luau. Tiki torches are a must and if you've got the money, splash out for a tiki bar, pig on a spit and some buff island men to serve you. If you are on a tighter budget, decorate with inexpensive bamboo reeds and palms.

Fake leis are available at most dollar stores, but if you can afford it then treat yourselves to real flower ones or have the guests make their own leis with flower and string. Grass skirts are readily available on the Internet and, if you aren't too shy, try a coconut top. For those who are more modest, a bikini top or even Hawaiian print shirt will do.

If you aren't able or interested in putting a pig on a spit, there are still lots of great foods to serve at your luau. Fish or seafood are obvious main dishes or Teriyaki beef or chicken are also good choices. Serve up sides of potato salad, spinach salad and baked sweet potatoes. For dessert, make a large fruit platter of pineapple, papaya, melon, strawberries, or mango – basically whatever you like and can get at your local grocer.

Serve your drinks in coconuts and have lots of little drink umbrellas. Mai Tai's and Piña Colada's are popular Hawaiian drinks that really pack a punch so consider having a few virgin versions available, too.

Hula Hooping is a fun activity and you can have a competition to see who can go the longest or do the best tricks. Hula is the traditional Hawaiian dance, so hire an instructor or check out how-to videos online and get those hips swinging!

Aloha!

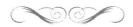

"A day without laughter is a day wasted."

~ Charlie Chaplin

Down the Rabbit Hole
YouTube favorites night

There are lots of funny clips on YouTube, many of which you will have been forwarded in the past. Ask everyone to pick the one they love the most and then just open up the laptop and share. If you have an HDMI cable and your laptop and TV are compatible, you can set it up so everyone can watch on the TV while someone drives the laptop.

The game starts with your favorites, but then you view suggested clips on your favorite's page…and then the suggested clips for those clips and-on-and-on "down the rabbit hole". You end up seeing some really funny and random stuff… Don't be surprised when a few hours have gone by in a flash!

In case you don't have any favorites, here are a few suggestions on good places to start:

1. Cheap flights with subtitles
2. Louis CK - Everything's amazing and nobody's happy
3. Battle at Kruger National Park

1. http://www.youtube.com/watch?v=HPyl2tOaKxM
2. http://www.youtube.com/watch?v=LU8DDYz68kM

Trivia Night

Team: __Master Minds__

Q1. When?
Answer __Saturday Night__

Q2. Where?
Answer __My Place__

Q3. Who?
Answer __Teams of up to 6__

Q4. Cost?
Answer __Completely free__

TOTAL ___

Trivial Pursuits

Just how clever is your crew? Find out with a competitive quiz night.

Trivia nights are great fun, especially when you get a group of super-competitive friends to participate. Instead of going out for one and over-paying for booze and food, you can easily host a trivia night in your own home.

Once you've decided whom to invite and have received all your RSVPs you can decide how many teams to have. The best way to assign teams is for the host to randomly pull names out of a hat on the evening. The host of the event is responsible for reading the questions and keeping tally of the scores, in addition to coming up with all of the questions or organizing a questions package. The questions are extremely important, as they will set the mood of the evening.

As a rule, you should plan for seven rounds of ten questions, which will last anywhere from two-and-a-half to four hours. A great way to break down the rounds is to give each one a different theme, which will also make coming up with the questions easier if you don't plan to buy a questions package.

Yet another variation on this is to have each guest write down ten trivia questions specifically about themselves, their lives, or their families – this is a great way to get to know each other better!

Each team will need an answer sheet for each round. At the end of the round, team captains submit their answers to the host who then tallies up the scores. A scoreboard is a great way to keep the competition intense and you can easily make one with a bit of poster board.

If you have the budget for it, get prizes for the winning team. If not, bragging rights for the winners will usually suffice!

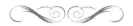

"Give me books, French wine, fruit, fine weather and a little music played out of doors by somebody I do not know."

~ John Keats

Uncork a Book

*Pop over to a friend's to pair and share your
favorite reads and reds…or whites!*

This is a fun literary get-together that allows friends to introduce each other to good books and good wines. Everyone brings their favorite book paired with a bottle of their favorite wine and has a chance to tell everyone what they love about each. You will find that some of your tastes are very similar and you can introduce each other to different authors and new wineries!

A twist on this event is for everyone to bring a recipe and wine (or other drink) from a meal described in their book. Or, if you really want to immerse yourselves in another world for an evening, take it one step further by dressing as the literary characters.

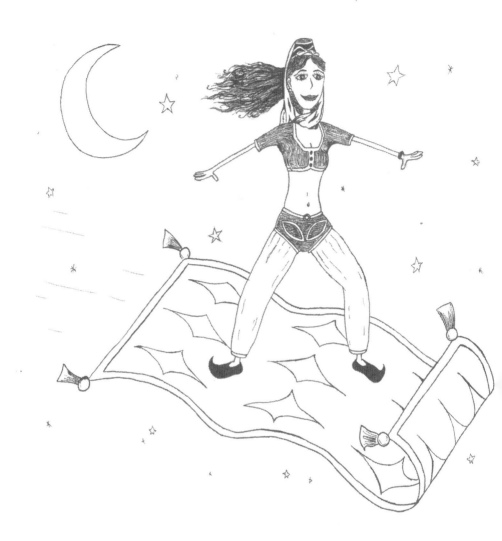

Moroccan Fantasy

*Take a magic carpet ride to exotic Morocco
for your own Arabian Night.*

The warm months are best for eating on the floor outside surrounded by brightly colored pillows, linens and stamped lanterns. If you have a hookah, or know someone who does, they make a great centerpiece.

Start your culinary adventure to Morocco with roasted eggplant accompanied by a yogurt dish and olives with harissa. Rock the Kasbah with exotic flavors of Moroccan lamb cooked in a tajine, which is an earthenware pot that cooks the meat to perfection, served with side dishes of couscous and chickpea salad. Make sure to provide plenty of khobz, which is Moroccan bread, as Moroccans eat with their hands and the proper way to eat Moroccans food is to scoop it up with khobz.

No Moroccan meal would be complete without Moroccan Mint Tea or Arabic Coffee. While Morocco is an Islamic state, alcohol is widely available in many Moroccan cities, like Casablanca, and there are a few Moroccan beer brands that you maybe able to find at specialty spirit stores.

End the evening by giving each other henna tattoos on your hands, wrists, ankles and feet and then, if you aren't too full, try a little belly dancing!

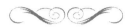

*"Just play.
 Have fun.
  Enjoy the game."*

~ Michael Jordan

Wii Love to Compete

Multi-player video game competition

Whether you've got a PlayStation, Wii, or Xbox, there are so many different kinds of games and you can choose from dance competitions, pub games, beach sports…the options abound. Be as elaborate as you want with round-robin tournaments or basic elimination events.

If you and the gals are keen to get into shape, then fire up the Wii Fit Plus and see who has the best level of fitness. Set goals for yourselves and in a few weeks get together again to see how you're tracking.

Be sure to have plenty of easy-to-eat foods 🍴 on hand or the pizza guy's number close by and play into the night!

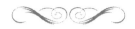

Popular Herbs

Herb	Light	Height	Type
Basil	Sun, Part-sun	1-3 feet	Annual
Chamomile	Sun, Part-sun	6-24 inches	Annual, Perennial
Chives	Sun, Part-sun	8-18 inches	Perennial
Cilantro, coriander	Sun, Part-sun	5-24 inches	Annual
Dill	Sun	1-3 feet	Annual
Lemongrass	Sun, Part-sun	3-6 feet	Perennial
Mint	Sun, Part-sun	1-4 feet	Perennial
Oregano	Sun	1-2 feet	Perennial
Parsley	Sun	8-24 inches	Annual
Rosemary	Sun	1-6 feet	Perennial
Sage	Sun, Part-sun	1-2 feet	Perennial
Tarragon	Sun, Part-sun	1-5 feet	Perennial
Thyme	Sun	3-12 inches	Perennial

Green-thumb Gathering

Get together and grow your own herb gardens.

Herbs add flavor to lots of recipes. After this night you'll have your own window box overflowing with fresh herbs that you can dip into whenever you need! This is a fun way of saving money in the long run by planting your own miniature herb garden. And you're doing your bit for the environment to boot.

Everything you need can be found in the larger department stores or (even better) support your local garden center and get tons of free advice, too. Buy each guest a window box and pick up potting mix and a variety of herbs such as; basil, mint, parsley, dill, chives, rosemary, sage…All these herbs can be grown from seed or for a quick fix you can buy a starter plant. You can always ask each person to chip in for what you have purchased or have everyone bring their own supplies. Arrange the bits and pieces you need, crack open a bottle of wine or down a wheatgrass shot and get gardening!

Many herb plants are sold in little containers ready to go, but be sure not to plant too many herbs in one window box. Remind your guests to water regularly and ensure that their herbs get plenty of sunlight.

As an added bonus you could print up some recipes that involve fresh herbs to provide your guests with culinary inspiration for their new herb garden, or make it a dinner party and have each guest bring a dish that includes one of your herbs.

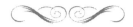

"Summer afternoon - summer afternoon; to me those have always been the two most beautiful words in the English language."

~ Henry James

Sizzlin' Summer Soiree

A BBQ & pool party is a great way to cool off over the summer and have some fun in the sun.

Even if you don't have a pool you can make your own summer shindig in a backyard or rooftop terrace with inflatable pools, which can be even more fun. Real pool or blow-up pool, all you need are a few toys and some good friends for a hot day of cool fun. Have everyone bring squirt guns, swimming noodles, and don't forget the rafts - a must have!

There are lots of fun games to get everyone in the pool if you've got one. Marco Polo is easy and free, but you'll need to get a net and ball for a game of water polo. Diving for items such as rings, sticks, or coins is always fun and you can have competitions to see who can collect them all the quickest. If they're in season, grease up a watermelon with some lard, throw it in the deep end and see which of your guests can get it to the edge the fastest.

BBQ foods like hotdogs, hamburgers and salads are simple to prepare and cook. Lemonade and ice tea are refreshing drinks when you're out in the sun and an ice-cold beer is the perfect match for a BBQ.

Most importantly, don't forget to Slip, Slap, Slop!

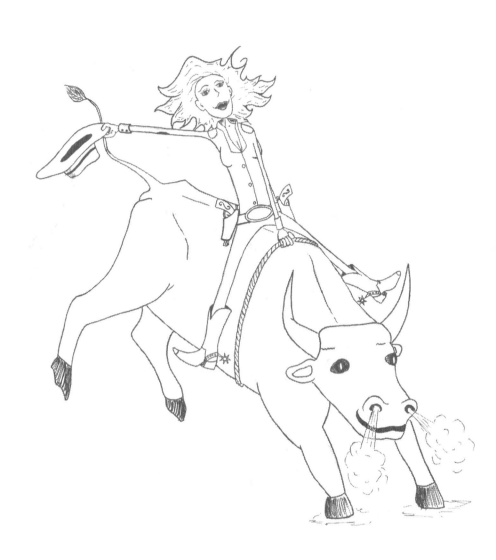

Wild West Hoedown

Have your pardners mosey on over fer some boot stompin' fun!

Y'all are bound to have a great night when you giddyup on over to a home on the range for a good old-fashion Wild West hoedown! To make it look like the west outline your party space with painted cardboard cactus cutouts and use western table clothes with tiny hay bails. You can get the straw at most craft stores. Decorate with lassos and bandanas and hang wanted posters made with pictures of all your outlaw guests.

Ask everyone to dress for the west as cowgirls and for chow serve-up some chilli 🍴 and beer. Tune into the Country Music channel or download some Johnny Cash to set the mood. Kick up your heels with some line dancing and if none of you know how, hire a pro or watch a video on-line to show you how to dance the Boot Scootin Boogie.

A really fun game is a bicycle rodeo, which just involves setting up obstacles in the backyard and racing around them on bicycles, or the kids trikes if you have yung uns. If you don't have the space for a rodeo, a lasso contest with stuffed sheep or other stuffed animals is also a real hoot! For those with a big budget, hire a mechanical bull!

This rootin' tootin' jamboree will have all the cowgirls hollerin' "yee-haw"!

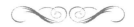

"Bear in mind three essential qualities in all games of intellect: Never to show selfishness or to wound the feelings of your adversary. To be modest with a good game. To lose without ill-temper, and to win without bragging."

~ W. Patterson

Promise You Won't Be Board Game Night

Board games are never boring when played with a few good friends!

There are hundreds of board games to choose from and your choice should depend on the mood and tone you want to set for the evening. If you just want to relax and test your intellect, then choose a game like Boggle, Scrabble, or Trivial Pursuit. If you want to get a bit livelier then games like Cranium, Taboo or Sorry! are sure to spice it up a bit (and if you're looking to get a little wild, incorporate drinking penalties into the rules).

Between you and your friends you should have a choice of several board game options. No matter what games you chose, you are in for a fun night when you get your game on with friends. You will really get to know each other when the competition heats up!

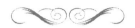

Progressive Dinner Sample Schedule

6:00-6:45pm	Cocktails and canapés	Lorna's
6:45-7:30pm	Soups & salads	Sarah's
7:30-8:30pm	Main course	Lisa's
8:30-late	Dessert	Kim's

Guest and dish/drink list

1. Lorna (hostess 1) - Chicken skewers, Pineapple cheese ball
2. Sarah (hostess 2) - Waldorf salad, Strawberry soup
3. Lisa (hostess 3) - Roast
4. Kim (hostess 4) - Cheese platter, wine
5. Megan - Pre-mixed cocktail
6. Samantha - Garlic bread, 2 bottles wine
7. Heather - Greenbean casserole, 1 bottle wine
8. Christi - Roast veggies, 1 bottle wine
9. Malee - Garlic and rosemary mashed potatoes, 1 bottle wine
10. Laura - Fruit platter, 1 bottle wine

Progressive Dinner

Instead of asking "My house or yours?" why not do "My house THEN yours"?

Progressive Dinners (also known as Safari Suppers in the UK) are a fun way to share the responsibility of a dinner party by having each course prepared and eaten at a different host's house.

Plan a maximum of four courses and allow for 45 minutes to an hour at each home. Courses could be Cocktails and Canapés, Starters (such as soups and salads), Main course (including side dishes), and Dessert (including sweets, cheese plates, coffee and after dinner drinks). To keep it fair, have guests whose homes are not being visited provide the drinks or a dish for one of the courses.

Ideally you will go to houses that are within close proximity of each other (preferably walking distance if you plan to drink). Otherwise, make sure you have a few sober drivers, one sober driver with a large van, or arrange maxi-taxis or a limo service if you've got the budget.

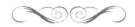

"The things I want to know are in books; my best friend is the man who'll get me a book I ain't read."

~ Abraham Lincoln

Hardback, paperback, do you want this book back?

Avoid library late fees by booking in a night with friends to swap some good reads.

With books costing around $30 this is an inexpensive way to get a few great books to read with the bonus of an endorsement from a friend who has read the book.

Ask all of your guests to bring at least three books that they have read and enjoyed. As your guests arrive, have them sign in and list their book titles and then organize books by genre and alphabetize by author's surname, just like at a bookstore. Once the shelves are stacked you can open your shop and invite everyone to start browsing!

As some guests may eventually want their books returned, the hostess should keep track of who is taking which book on the sign-in sheet. Also, make sure those who want their books back put their names in the front.

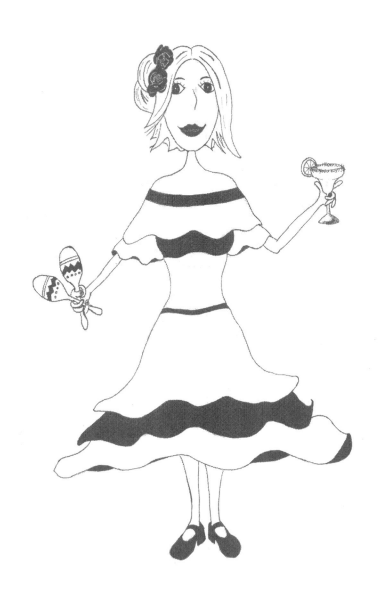

Mexican Fiesta

Señoritas don your ponchos and sombreros
for a Mexican Fiesta.

Get out the Margarita glasses and decorate your pad with Mexican flags and sombreros to create a real Mexican feel. Ice down some Corona's and wedge up some limes, which you may also need for tequila shots.

Chips and salsa, tacos and burritos are all obvious food choices, but if you want to try authentic Mexican cuisine there are a range of recipes online. Also, don't forget about dessert - churros or fried ice cream are great choices.

If you want to get a little wild, get a piñata and serve up some tequila (just make sure it's the good stuff, not the rubbish with a worm that guarantees a massive hangover). If you've got the cash, get a tequila donkey!

Olé!

 http://www.mexgrocer.com/mexican-recipes.html

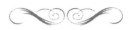

"I had always thought that once you grew up you could do anything you wanted - stay up all night or eat ice cream straight out of the container."

~ Bill Bryson

Ice Cream Sundays

I scream, you scream, we all scream for ice cream!

Sundays are great days for creating an ice cream parlor where guests can serve their own ice cream sundaes. ♫ Upon arrival, let everyone decorate their own old-fashioned paper soda jerk hats with their names on them. If you've got the budget and the time, have aprons for each girl to decorate with white and pink polka dots and an appliqué of an ice cream cone.

If you or any of your friends have special ice cream sundae dishes, these would add to the authenticity of your ice cream parlor; otherwise, normal bowls will suffice. Also, you will need a metal tub or cooler with ice to keep the ice cream and whipped cream cold.

Put out all of the ingredients in a buffet and let your guests make their own delicious creations. Basic flavors of ice cream to have on hand include vanilla, chocolate and strawberry, but if you are having a lot of guests or have more sophisticated taste buds there plenty of fancy flavors to choose from (to speed up the process and save on the mess consider putting one person in charge of the ice cream scoops).

Ask each guest to bring two of her favorite toppings, but make sure you know what everyone is bringing beforehand so you don't double-up; sprinkles, chocolate and peanut butter chips, chopped nuts, shredded coconut, M&M's, fruit in syrup and maraschino cherries are just a few suggestions. Don't forget the sauces: butterscotch, caramel, chocolate, strawberry... Finally, dessert liqueurs such as Bailey's Irish Cream and Kahlua also taste great on ice cream!

Dip-in and enjoy!

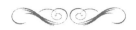

Birthstones

Month	Stone	Symbolization
January	Garnet	Constancy, true friendship and fidelity
February	Amethyst	Sincerity and peace of mind
March	Aquamarine Bloodstone	Courage, victory and confidence
April	Diamond	Innocence
May	Emerald	Love, success
June	Pearl Alexandrite	Health, longevity
July	Ruby	Contentment
August	Peridot	Married happiness
September	Sapphire	Clear thinking
October	Opal Tourmaline	Hope
November	Topaz	Fidelity
December	Turquoise Zircon	Prosperity

Be Dazzling

Bling the girls up with your own unique jewelry designs.

Got any lonely necklaces? Turn them into a set by making a pair of matching earrings! It's a fun simple way to jazz up your collection. And with the necklaces providing a design template, even the least creative of us can come up with earrings to match. If you don't have any necklaces that you are looking to turn into a set, Google jewelry design ideas to find other jewelry making projects.

Jewelry making supplies for beginners are pretty basic so don't go running out to the craft store and spending heaps of money on numerous packets of wires, beads, rhinestones, clasps and tools. The basic supplies that you will need are jewelry wire, beads and findings (head pins, clasps, ear wires or posts and ear clutches). The basic tools are a flush cutter, round nose pliers, chain nose and bent nose tools. There are plenty of jewelry making kits that contain all of these necessary supplies, so have one ready for each of your guests or ask them to bring their own. If you're really low on cash, you could all pool together for one set and share.

You'll enjoy showing off your fabulous new baubles, all the more special because you made them yourselves.

Alternatively, have someone who does home-jewelry parties come to your house with their wares.

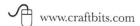
www.craftbits.com

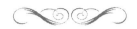

Queen of Hearts: *Curtsy while you're thinking. It saves time.*

Alice: [curtsying] *Yes, Your Majesty, but I just wanted to ask you...*

Queen of Hearts: *I'll ask the questions! Do you play croquet?*

Alice: *Why, yes, Your Majesty.*

Queen of Hearts: *Then let the game begin!*

- from ***Alice's Adventures in Wonderland***
written by Lewis Carroll

Croquet, anyone?

*Ladies on the lawn sipping tea and playing croquet...
how very civilized?*

Croquet lawn parties are the perfect way to greet the warmer weather and they are also a great time to get your best whites out of the back of the closet.

Guests should be served an iced beverage upon arrival. A light lunch of finger sandwiches (cucumber, egg and cress, smoked salmon) can be served while guests are mingling, too.

The set-up of croquet is very basic and only requires an open space and a croquet set, which includes two stakes, nine wickets and a couple of mallets and balls. If you and your friends don't own a set, chances are good that someone's parents or grandma have one hidden away in the garage or shed. The aim of the game is to get your color ball through all the wickets. The basic rules of croquet are fairly simple and if you don't know them you can easily download them from the Internet.

With all of your friends together on a sunny afternoon you are sure to have a wicked good time with the wickets!

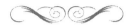

Simple Savings Tips

1. Make your own coffee
2. Bottle your own water
3. Brew your own beer
4. Cook at home at least five days a week
5. Plan your meals for the week and make a shopping list
6. Grocery shop with a list
7. Buy in bulk
8. Buy generic brands
9. Avoid ATM fees
10. Take public transport instead of driving whenever possible

Dollars & Sense Dinner

*Fight the urge to splurge while sharing
a potluck feast and financial tips.*

While some of us are very good with our money, others struggle to save, get ahead or even make ends meet. Most of us have at least one frugal friend who could teach us a thing or two about making better financial decisions while still having fun. If your group is full of females who are notorious for not taking control of their financial security, consult the websites of Suze Orman or Smart Money to get a few ideas on the best way to empower yourselves and take control of your finances.

You can all share tips on ways to save money on your weekly shopping, places to buy good quality clothes and cosmetics at a discount, coupon sites that can help you save on brands you already buy, and other tips on where you have been able to find good bargains recently.

Have a potluck feast where everyone brings a favorite dish that cost less that $10 to prepare. For drinks, see who can find the best bottle of wine for under $8.

Organize a Goals Group and have everyone set a goal (whether it be to get out of debt, save the deposit for a first home, or take a trip-of-a lifetime). Support each other in achieving them by setting milestones and deadlines, with monthly check-ins.

www.suzeorman.com
www.smartmoney.com

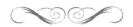

"Nothing makes you more tolerant of a neighbor's noisy party than being there."

~ Franklin P. Jones

Howdy, neighborini!

Block party to meet the women on your street.

Invite the women on your street or in your unit block over to get to know them better. Block parties are great to do any time, but are particularly good if you are new to the area, have started working from home or have young children who you care for at home. Meeting new people who live close by can lessen feelings of isolation and you will be pleasantly surprised at how friendly people really are if you extend the hand of friendship first.

Decide how many people you would like to invite, will it just be women in your unit block, just mums, just women working from home or the entire street? Ensure you have the room and provisions to cater for them and if this is a major concern ask people to RSVP. Pop a little invite into each person's mailbox and include your contact details so people can get in touch without having to knock on the door.

Don't worry too much about preparing lots of food etc… Keep it simple with dips, nibbles and a maybe a glass of bubbly. Alternatively you may want to ask people to bring a plate of food to share and whatever they want to drink.

Have name tags ready! As the host you may need to take the lead and introduce people to each other or if you are new to the area you may find that people do this for you.

Finally, you could combine the party with fund-raising, where each guests makes a nominal donation to a local charity. This gives people a common purpose and not only are they meeting new people, but also making a difference. Be careful to keep the evening light and not to go on too much about the charity's plight (even if you are really passionate about it), as this can turn people off and you have to remember that these people are your neighbors and you will see them regularly!

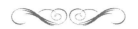

Popular Constellations

Name	Meaning	Hemisphere & Season
Andromeda	The Princess	Northern - autumn Southern - spring
Aquarius	The Water Bearer	Northern - autumn Southern - spring
Cancer	The Crab	Northern - spring Southern - autumn
Cassiopeia	The Queen	Northern - year-round
Crux incl. 'Southern Cross'	The Cross	Southern - year-round
Gemini	The Twins	Northern - winter Southern - summer
Leo	The Lion	Northern - spring Southern - autumn
Orion	The Hunter	Northern - winter Southern - summer
Sagittarius	The Archer	Northern - summer Southern - winter
Scorpius	The Scorpion	Northern - summer Southern - winter
Taurus	The Bull	Northern - winter Southern - summer
Ursa Major incl. 'Big Dipper'	Great Bear	Northern - year-round
Ursa Minor* incl. 'Little Dipper'	Little Bear	Northern - year-round

Star Gazing

Sick of watching the television? Enjoy a peaceful night of watching the stars instead!

Ever wanted to know more about the arrangement of the stars up above? What better way to learn a little more about astronomy than looking up on a clear night with friends?

Check your calendar to avoid the full moon, as it will make the night sky brighter and other stars more difficult to see. Also consult the weather channel to make sure the forecast is favorable.

The sky is full of interesting constellations, stars and planets that are visible to the naked eye. The back yard or rooftop terrace is a great place to star gaze on a clear night and all you need is a small pair of binoculars (many amateur astronomy websites say binoculars work fine, so don't worry about getting a telescope unless one of your friends already has one) and some star charts. The Sky & Telescope website has great Getting Started in Astronomy pamphlets for the Northern and Southern Hemispheres and contains tips, instructions, charts and maps available as a downloadable 10-page, black-and-white Adobe PDF file suitable for printing and photocopying.

If any of your friends has an iPhone, you can also download a constellation app, which identifies the stars and planets when you aim the phone at the sky.

As it often gets cooler in the evening, make sure everyone dresses warmly for a fun night of exploring distant planets and galaxies!

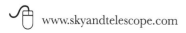
www.skyandtelescope.com

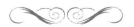

"Mystery is something that appeals to most everybody."

~ Angela Lansbury

WhoDunIt? Dinner

A murder mystery party that your guests will be dying to get into!

If you and your friends are bored to death with the same old dinner party, a Murder Mystery party is a killer idea that will liven up your evening. You can buy Murder Mystery kits at most stores that sell board games or just download one from the Internet. There are a wide variety of themes and you can decide how involved you want the plots to be and how many characters you will need to cast.

To properly execute your Murder Mystery party you will have to do a bit of planning. The kit instructions usually give ideas for decorations, menus, and costumes in addition to brief character bios and full character guides. Send out invitations at least three weeks before the night and ask everyone to RSVP within a week so you will know exactly how many guests will be playing. Make sure that everyone who plans to come will be there for the entire evening as late arrivals or early departures can ruin the game.

Cast the characters once you know exactly who is participating. At least a week before the night, send everyone some basic game info and their character guide so they can organize their costumes and start planning their act.

On the night, give everyone name tags to make remembering who's-who easier. Follow the instructions, which layout the plot line. After you figure out 'whodunit', hand out prizes for the best costumes, best detective, best actor and any other categories that are relevant to your game.

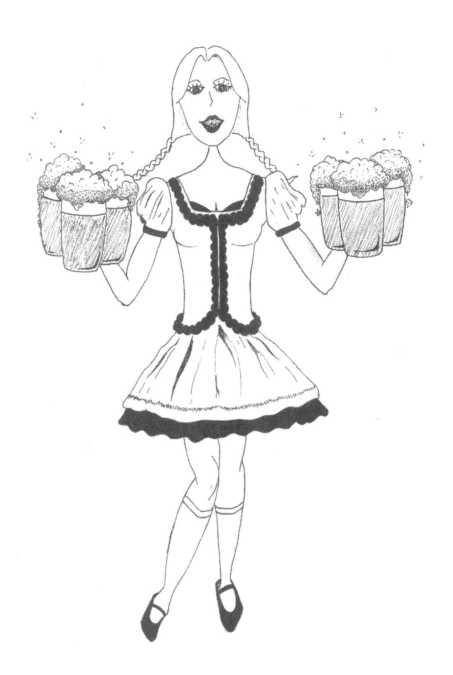

Oktoberfest

Willkommen to autumn!

When the leaves start to turn, download some Oompa music, decorate with a Bavarian theme, and don your lederhosen to celebrate Oktoberfest.

German beer is an essential ingredient to a genuine Oktoberfest celebration, but if all the Fräuleins aren't fond of the frothy brews then Riesling is a good authentic alternative. If it is cold for your Oktoberfest then serve Glühwein (pronounced glue-vine) a traditional German holiday drink. In addition to beer and/or wine, the menu should include pretzels, weiner schnitzel, German sausages, hot German potato salad, sauerkraut, and red cabbage. Black Forest cake is a must for dessert!

If you want to play a game and aren't worried about aggravating your neighbors, then have a yodelling contest to see who can yodelay-hee-hoo the best.

Prost!

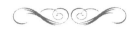

"There's just something about a fondue pot that invites conversation. Invites laughter. Invites coming together."

~ from The Melting Pot website
(www.meltingpot.com)

Fondue You Want to Come Over for Dinner?

A melting pot of fun new dinner experiences.

Fondue is a traditional Swiss dish of melted cheese served in a communal pot. However, since the 1950's fondue has come to include any sweet or savory food that is dipped into a hot pot of liquid.

For your fondue party, you can start with a cheese fondue followed by entrées including a variety of steak, chicken and seafood accompanied by homemade dipping sauces and vegetables. Finish up with fruit, marshmallows and biscuits with milk, white and dark chocolate or caramel fondue.

You can buy or hire a fondue set and it is best to have between four and six friends to one pot, with each person having a different color fondue fork.

Zodiac Quiz

Q1. If your birthday is March 21, what is your sign?
Answer <u>Aries</u>

Q2. What is the symbol for Libra?
Answer <u>Scales</u>

Q3. What are the water signs?
Answer <u>Cancer, Scorpio, Pisces</u>

Q4. Which sign is the Twins?
Answer <u>Gemini</u>

TOTAL ___

Hey baby, what's your sign?
The stars will align for a fun and enchanting evening of astrology.

People who aren't into astrology often have no clue about it and think it's just about their sun sign, and nothing more. Well tonight is your chance to dig a little deeper.

Decorate with a mystical theme: a zodiac chart; Chinese lanterns; animals that relate to the Chinese New Year; printed photos of astrological signs; moon, star and comet cutouts. You can also enhance the mystic ambiance by lighting incense and/or candles around the house.

Start off by testing your guests' knowledge of the zodiac. Create a short quiz with 10 questions to see how much they know about the zodiac signs.

If you've got the time and energy, have each of your guests send you their date, time, and place of birth a few days before the party and prepare charts for them beforehand, printing a summary version for them to take home. If not, you can pick up a copy of *The Birthday Book*, and give each friend an impromptu mini-reading.

Or, if you have the funds, hire an astrologer to give you an overview of the current astrological energies and also do mini-private readings (15 to 20 minutes each) to highlight the key elements of the birth chart for each party guest.

We all love hearing about ourselves (well, most of us anyway), so even friends who do not really believe in astrology should have fun hearing about their birth charts, signs, and the future events that could potentially happen in their lives. Even the most cynical friends should enjoy participating in this mystical evening.

 http://www.thesecretlanguageofbirthdays.com/

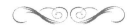

"Properly practiced, knitting soothes the troubled spirit, and it doesn't hurt the untroubled spirit either."

~ Elizabeth Zimmermann

Stitch N' Bitch

*With a simple pattern, needles and yarn
y'all will be in stitches.*

In the 21st Century knitting has become a hot trend with celebrities the likes of Cameron Diaz and Dakota Fanning jumping on the bandwagon. Knitting is no longer an old-fashioned activity reserved for grandmas and a night of knitting with your friends is a fun way to learn.

The tools you will need to get started include: yarn, knitting needles, a sewing needle, a pair of scissors and a crochet hook. Have someone who is an experienced knitter teach you the basic skills, such as: making a slip knot and casting on, forming the knit stitch, forming the purl stitch, casting off. If no one in your group knows how to knit, invite a capable mother or grandmother.

It is a good idea to start with a simple pattern such as a scarf or pot-holder and then graduate to more difficult patterns and techniques at each meeting. Instant-gratification knitting is a new trend where designers now offer patterns that can be knitted quickly on large needles, so find one of those patterns and see if you can each whip out a scarf on the night.

If you find you really enjoy knitting, then make a club! Pick a time and date (the first Tuesday of the month, for example, will make it easy for everyone to remember) and rotate the location to a different member's home each month. After a few months you may be able to start and finish a pattern in one evening and leave with your creation.

Knitting is a very relaxing hobby and can be quite therapeutic, especially when you are doing it with friends while having a good yarn!

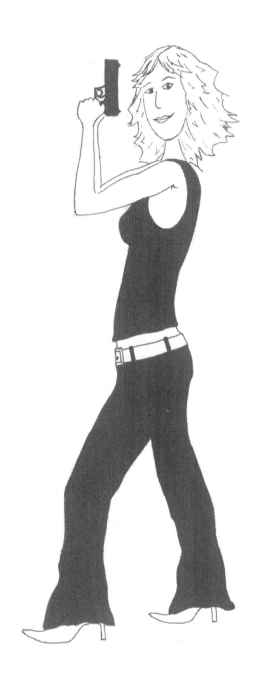

Bond Girls

Your mission, should you choose to accept it, is to throw a top-secret Secret Agent party.

Intel for this party can be disseminated as a code that includes the location, date, time and other important information relevant for your mission.

Tell your fellow agents that their mission is to disguise themselves as either an infamous Secret Agent or to create a new identity and go deep undercover.

There are many decor options for your evening of intrigue. If you are into Austin Powers, the Spy who Shagged Me, than you could re-create the Electric Psychedelic Pussycat Swingers Club and have shagadelic evening. If James Bond is more your thing then a swanky "Casino Royale" and place black silhouette targets around the party room (see page 43 for ideas on setting up a casino).

Play music from popular spy movies like, Totally Spies, Mission Impossible, Charlie's Angels, James Bond, Sherlock Holmes, etc. ♫

Serve your martinis shaken or stirred and don't forget….oh behave!

Godspeed agents.

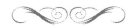

"I think we should just be friends...."

~ Any woman wanting to end a relationship...

Side-dishes and Left-overs for Dinner

Help your single girlfriends find a date.

If you or any of your friends are single and looking for pre-screened and available men, then this night is for you! Host a casual party where everyone brings either a single male friend (side-dish) or ex-boyfriend (left-over, one who you are still friends with but aren't interested in dating and you don't have feelings for each other any more). This night is also known as a "used-date" party, which was popularized on an episode of *Sex and the City*.

Even if you are married or in a relationship and don't have many straight guy friends, your partners are bound to have a few eligible single friends that could be a good match for one of your single girlfriends.

Regardless of whether you are bringing your 'side dishes' or 'leftovers', it may be best to not tell them about your ulterior motives, as it can feel a bit awkward if they know that you are trying to set them up. Just tell them you are getting a great group together so you can all meet some cool new people.

And, you never know, one woman's cast-off could be another woman's treasure!

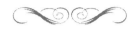

Popular Scents

Scent	Uses	Effects
Cedar	relieve anxiety and quell anxiety, irritation and fear	stimulating, elevating and opening
Cinnamon	faintness, weakness, depression, nervous exhaustion	improve mood, vigor and concentration
Eucalyptus	purification, health, healing, relieves headaches	revitalising, stimulating effect on the nervous system
Lavender	treat headaches, nervous tension, depression, sorrow and grief	induce peaceful sleep and increase feelings of well being
Mint	stimulate circulation, the heart and boost intellect and memory	soothing and stimulating effect on the brain
Orange	aid with nervousness, epileptic fits, melancholia and depression	relaxation, regeneration and calming down
Rose	increase concentration, regulate the appetite and overcoming obesity	creates a feeling of calm, well-being and in some, even happiness
Vanilla	depression, sorrow, and grief	warming, cheering, uplifting

Aroma-rama

Alter your mood, and possibly your health, while you sit back and smell the fragrances.

Aromatherapy is a trendy alternative medical therapy that uses essential oils and other aromatics to affect mood and promote health.

One of the most therapeutic aspects of aromatherapy is creating your own essential oil blends, which include aromatic and therapeutic blends. Aromatic blends are made solely for the enjoyment of their fragrance; while therapeutic blends can be made for emotional and physical wellbeing, beauty, skin care and hygiene. The Internet has heaps of information on aromatherapy including recipes, guides to essential oils, and useful articles.

Do it yourselves with a little on-line research; make a list of the oils, equipment and accessories required and then divide the list and assign items for each guest to bring. If that all sounds like too much work, it can be just as easy and inexpensive to find an aromatherapy consultant to come give you instruction on how to make the blends and who can provide you (at a cost, of course) with quality essentials oils, oil burners and accessories.

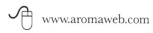 www.aromaweb.com

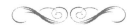

"That's the thing with handmade items. They still have the person's mark on them, and when you hold them, you feel less alone."

~ Aimee Bender

Card It Up Catch-up

Put this card-making night on the cards in the lead up to Christmas, or any time of year.

It is always nice to have a variety of greeting cards stashed for birthdays, baby and bridal showers, or when you just want to send a nice card to a friend. The thought and effort put into handmade cards mean so much more to their recipients than store-bought ones, so why not make your own while spending some fun time with friends?

The basic products you will need include card stock (white or colored), glitter, paint, paintbrushes, stencils, markers and glue. If you want to get really fancy, you can get embossing powders, cutting and embossing tools, adhesives and other embellishments at a craft supply store. If you or any of your friends are into scrapbooking, then you can easily use the tools and supplies you already own for your card making. Make a list of the supplies you will need and ask your guests to bring along any items you are missing or any special supplies that they would like to use and share.

If you are looking for some inspiration or ideas for your card making night, Martha Stewart's website has a Card-Making Center with heaps of card ideas for every occasion. There is a wide range of techniques and you can go as simple or elaborate as you like.

Serve season-appropriate foods and drinks (eggnog or mulled wine at Christmas) and enjoy time together making beautiful cards.

 www.marthastewart.com

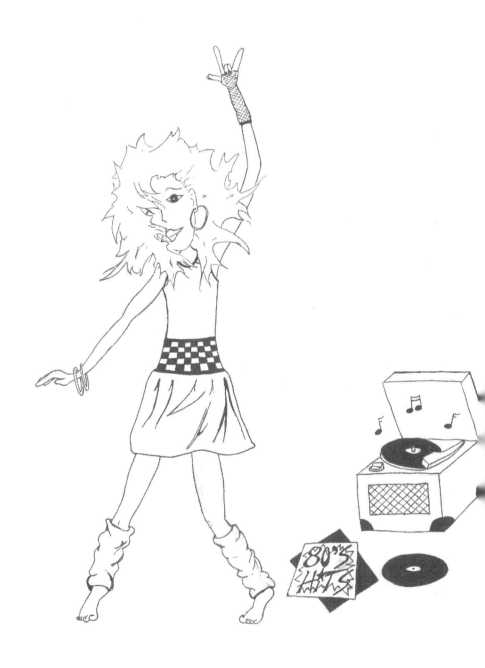

Girls Just Wanna Have Fun
80's Pop party

Dig deep into the back of your closets for those old jean jackets and leg warmers, pull out the crimping iron and ask the Valley Girls to Walk Like an Egyptian over to your pad for an 80's Pop party!

A strobe light and fog machine on the space you create for your dance floor will be totally radical. You can also decorate with 80's movie and music posters, easily found on eBay. Cut neon posters into geometric shapes and hang them on the walls and watch them glow when you turn on the blue light.

If you don't have clothes left over from the 80's (or the fashion-disaster of the late 2000's), head out to Good Will or Vinnie's and look for anything neon or short and puffy. Outfit ideas include:

- A big sweatshirt with the neck cut out hanging off one shoulder with a big belt low on your hips over peg-legged acid-washed jeans screams Mall Rat.
- Leotard and tights, knit leg warmers and athletic headband and wrist warmers – think Olivia Newton John.
- Black mesh tank, short skirt, and leggings with a bunch of bracelets over lace fingerless gloves, dangly earrings and a big bow on top of wild hair makes the best Material Girl get-up.
- Other ideas are Punky Brewster, punk rock chick, or for anyone a little older – The Golden Girls. Don't forget glow necklaces!

Lots of food critics dis 80's cuisine, but it would be legit to serve tri-colored pasta salad, Spaghetti O's, potato skins and quiches. And, like, Omigod it would be totally awesome if you served Fuzzy Navels 🍸 and wine coolers!

If you've still got it, break out the boom box and your old 80's cassette tapes. If not, just put together a playlist. Either way it's time to get loose, Footloose!

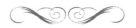

"C is for Cookie, that's good enough for me."

~ Cookie Monster

Cookie Exchange

Who stole the cookie from the cookie jar? You won't care when you bring home four-dozen cookies!

Got lots of holiday baking to do? Hosting a cookie exchange is a nice break from the stress of the 'silly season' and allows you to get dozens of different kinds of cookies while only having to bake one recipe.

As calendars fill up quickly during silly season, plan your party in the early part of December and send out invitations a month in advance. Ask all of your guests to RSVP ASAP so that you know what type of cookies everyone will be baking and can avoid duplicate recipes.

Request that cookies are baked at least a day before the exchange as freshly baked cookies can be quite fragile and difficult to transport. Furthermore, it will reduce stress on the day and no-shows due to running out of time to bake. Hangovers can be quite common during silly season and if anyone wakes up with one on the day of the cookie exchange and hasn't already baked four-dozen cookies, they aren't likely to make it (we're not saying we're speaking from experience, but trust us on this one!).

Cookies should be arranged on a platter or in a cookie tin or basket and everyone should bring a large container to carry away swapped cookies. On the day, have everyone put their cookies on the swapping table and serve canapés with some spiked eggnog or mulled wine. After everyone arrives and has had some sips and nibbles, gather around the swapping table with your containers and take turns introducing your cookies. Start the cookie swap by going around the table taking 4 cookies from each platter.

After the swap is complete guest can start sampling the cookies or save them all to take home to share with their families and holiday guests.

Perfect Match

Guest: <u>Laura</u>
Partner: <u>Ian</u>

Q1. What is your favorite alcoholic beverage (be specific)?
Answer: <u>Beer - Stella Artois</u>

Q2. What is your favorite appetizer?
Answer: <u>Buffalo Wings</u>

Q3. What was your childhood nickname?
Answer: <u>Foogie</u>

Q4. What is your maternal grandma's name?
Answer: <u>Bernadette</u>

Q5. How old were you when you got your first cell phone?
Answer: <u>20</u>

Q6. What is your greatest fear?
Answer: <u>Being stuck in a small space</u>

Q7. What was the last book you read?
Answer: <u>Unplayable</u>

Perfect Match

*Find out how well you know your partners
with a personal quiz night.*

Everyone thinks they know their partner well, but dig a little deeper and it can be surprising what they don't know. Compete against your friends in a series of revealing question rounds to determine who knows (and doesn't know) their partner best. If the gals are all single, then partner everyone up and see how well you know your buddies!

At least a week before the night, the hostess sends a list of revealing questions to all of the guests' partners. The hostess can come up with four rounds of seven questions, or have all of the guests submit two or three questions if it's too difficult to come up with all the questions on their own. Partners must return their answers in a sealed envelope to the hostess.

Make sure four of the questions are the partner's favorite appetizer, beer, wine and cocktail. Instead of the host catering, have guests bring what they think is their partner's favorite appetizer and beer, wine or cocktail (depending on what the guest wants to drink for the evening).

On the night, seat guests in a circle and give everyone an answer sheet for each round. The person to the left of each guest gets the sealed envelope of answers for the guest on her right. The host asks each question in the round allowing a few minutes for guests to write down her answers. Take a break after each round and let everyone score her neighbor. After the break go around the circle and have the guests share their answers and find out if they are right or wrong. Put the scores on a scoreboard and then start the next round; continue until all rounds are finished and the winners are decided.

Results could surprise you!

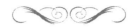

"Dress shabbily and they remember the dress; dress impeccably and they remember the woman."

~ Coco Chanel

Best Dressed

Fancy frock dress-up party

We all need to feel fancy once in awhile and what better way than with a decadent dress-up high tea. It is a shame that we only get to wear wedding and bridesmaids dresses once, and there so few occasions to wear ball gowns, so why not get them out of their garment bags and enjoy them once more?

If you have three-tiered cake stands and nice china, this is a great time to get them out! Indulge in delicious finger sandwiches, divine chocolates, cakes, and of course, scones with jam and cream.

Share stories and reminisce about the special moments spent in your dresses while sipping on a few selections of tea and/or a piccolo of champagne each if you feel like something bubbly.

Call each other darling, and be sure to keep those noses and pinkies up in the air!

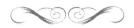

"Every great dream begins with a dreamer. Always remember, you have within you the strength, the patience, and the passion to reach for the stars to change the world."

~ Harriet Tubman

Reach for the Stars

What do you want to be when you grow up?

No matter what age we are, we've all got as-yet-unrealized goals and dreams and creating a vision board can help you achieve them. Have your friends bring a stack of magazines and provide everyone with a piece of cardboard or canvas. Some scissors, glue, and something to draw with are all the tools you need.

Then let your imaginations run wild and create collages that represent the things you still want out of life. They can be material goods, vacation destinations, or future career plans – anything goes when you're making a vision board!

Putting your goals on paper and creating images can help to cement them in your mind. More often than not, your subconscious will do the rest of the work and help you come up with solutions for achieving them you might never have imagined. Either way, you'll have fun sharing your visions with your friends. And you never know – someone there might be able to help you realize your dream – all you have to do is share it!

If you want to take your visions to the next level right away, organize a Goals Group and have everyone pick one of their goals. Support each other in achieving them by setting milestones and deadlines, with monthly check-ins.

 www.thesuccessprinciples.com/resources_index.php

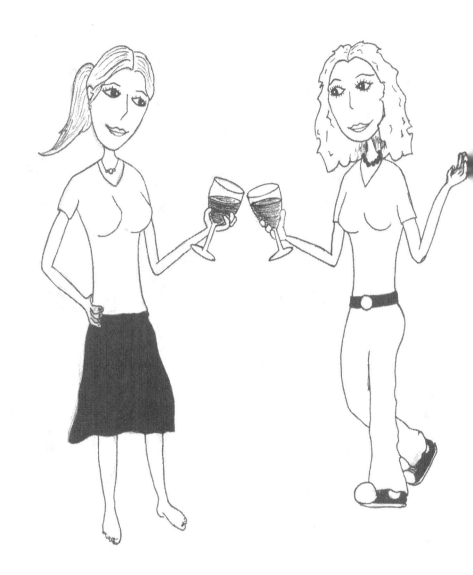

Wine Club

With over 150 commercially available wine varieties, you could keep this club going every month for over a decade!

This club is perfect if you have a few wine-enthusiast friends who are interested in learning more. Every month you can have wine club at a different person's house and the host can choose the variety of wine you will explore. Each guest will bring a bottle of the chosen variety.

Prepare everything before the guests arrive by putting out a communal spittoon and arranging seats for the wine tasting (each seat should have a notebook and pen, tasting glass and a glass of water). The hostess can provide hors d'oeuvres, or, have each guest bring a dish that matches their wine.

The hostess should do some research prior to the night and provide a little background on the grape variety to assist everyone in detecting the aromas and flavors in the wine. Next, everyone has a turn to present her wine and pour a tasting glass for all to examine the color, aroma and taste of each wine. Discuss.

Finally after tasting all the wines, and with palates somewhat impaired, attempt to do a blind tasting. Put each wine in a brown bag, taste one at a time and using your skills see whether you are able to tell which wine is which and write down your guesses. At this point it often gets a little rowdy as some people are certain of their impeccable palates and others become dismayed and confused. After the blind tasting reveal the order that the wines were poured and see whom the true connoisseurs really are!

 http://www.alexandramcguigan.blogspot.com.au

Drink Recipes

Mani, Pedi and Martini Party
French Martini

1 1/2 oz (375ml) Belvedere vodka, chilled
1/4 oz (125ml) Chambord or raspberry liqueur
1/4 oz (125ml) pineapple juice
Twist lemon peel

Place ice in a chilled cocktail shaker. Add the vodka, liqueur and juice and shake until well combined. Strain the vodka into the glasses and serve immediately with lemon peel.

Naughty or Nice Night
Topsy-Turvy

1 oz (295ml) dark rum
1 oz (295ml) light rum
1 oz (295ml) lemon-lime soda
Splash guava juice
Splash mango juice

Mix all ingredients in a glass over ice.
Serve with orange wedge garnish and umbrella.

Saturday Night Fever
Harvey Wallbanger

1 oz (295ml) vodka
1/2 oz (148ml) Galliano
4 oz (1 liter) orange juice
12 thin orange slices

Pour vodka and orange juice into a Collins glass over ice cubes and stir. Float Galliano on top and serve with an orange slice.

Spring Fling
Mint Julep

4 fresh mint sprigs
1 tsp powdered sugar

2 1/2 oz (740ml) bourbon whiskey
2 tsp water

Muddle mint leaves, powdered sugar, and water in a Collins glass. Fill the glass with crushed ice and add bourbon. Top with more crushed ice and garnish with a mint sprig.

Hawaiian Luau
Mai Tai

1 oz (295ml) light rum
1/2 oz o (148ml) orange curaçao
1/4 oz (75ml) orgeat syrup

juice from one fresh lime
1/4 oz (75ml) simple syrup
1/2 oz (148ml) dark rum

Pour all the ingredients except the dark rum into a shaker with ice cubes. Shake well. Strain into a Collins glass half filled with ice. Top with the dark rum. Serve with fresh fruit garnishes.

Croquet, anyone?
Southern Sweet Ice Tea

6 regular tea bags
2 cups boiling water
6 cups cold water

1/8 tsp baking soda
1.5 - 2 cups sugar

Sprinkle baking soda into a 64 ounce (2 liter), heat-proof, glass pitcher. Pour in boiling water, and add tea bags. Cover, and allow to steep for 15 minutes. Remove tea bags, and discard; stir in sugar until dissolved. Pour in cool water and chill in refrigerator.

Long Island Iced Tea

1 oz (295ml) vodka
1 oz (295ml) rum
1 oz (295ml) tequila
2 oz (590ml) cola

1 oz (295ml) gin
1 oz (295ml) triple sec liqueur
2 tsp orange juice
1 wedge lemon

In a cocktail mixer full of ice, combine vodka, gin, rum, triple sec and tequila. Add orange juice and cola. Shake vigorously until frothy. Strain into a tall glass filled with ice and garnish with wedge of lemon.

Oktoberfest
Glühwein

1 gallon (4 liters or roughly 5 bottles) red wine
Caster sugar (amount proportional to quality of red wine, the worse the wine the more sugar you need, add it to taste, but start with about 2 cups)
7 cinnamon sticks, halved
16 whole cloves
2 oranges
1 punnet berries (black are good)
10 (whole) allspice berries
2 cups of orange juice
Brandy, sweet sherry or port

Pour wine into a large pot on the stove over very low heat – do NOT boil! Cut the oranges into slices and insert 3 cloves into each slice and add to wine with cinnamon sticks and allspice. Add in the sherry or port and orange juice. Add in 2 cups of sugar and berries and stir. Stir occasionally for 30 minutes to allow spices to infuse, tasting frequently and adding sugar if needed. Simmer another 30 minutes.

Girls Just Wanna Have Fun
Fuzzy Navel

2 oz (590ml) peach schnapps
3 oz (887ml) peach brandy
1 1/2 oz (444ml) triple sec
Orange juice
Cherries

Mix schnapps, brandy and triple sec in a highball glass.
Fill with orange juice and ice to taste.
Garnish with cherries.

Food Recipes

Favorite Flicks Fest
Popcorn Balls

1 c white sugar
1/3 cup white corn syrup
3/4 tsp vanilla
1/2 cube (or stick) butter (2 oz / 56g)

3/4 tsp salt
1/3 cup water
3-4 quarts of popped corn

Combine all the ingredients except the vanilla and popped corn. Cook stirring until all the sugar is dissolved. Continue cooking without stirring until the syrup forms a brittle ball in cold water. Add vanilla and stir only enough to mix it through the hot syrup. Place the popped corn in a bowl large enough for mixing. Pour the cooked syrup slowly over the popped corn mix well. Keep hands wet to form the balls.

Roll Out the Red Carpet
Pineapple Cheese Ball

2 x 8 oz (225g) blocks cream cheese
2 Tbsp chopped green pepper
2 Tbsp chopped white part of green onion
1 small can crushed pineapple (drained)
2 tsp seasoned salt
2 x 1 cup chopped pecans

Mix together all ingredients but 1 cup chopped pecans. Roll into a ball and roll in second cup chopped pecans.

Moroccan Fantasy
Khobz

2 cups whole-wheat flour
1/4 cup sesame seeds
1/2 tsp sugar
1/2 Tbsp dry active yeast

1 tsp anise seeds
1/2 tsp salt
2 Tbsp extra-virgin olive oil
1.5 cups warm water

Use your hands to mix together the flour, salt, anise seeds, sesame seeds, sugar and yeast. Slowly add the olive oil and warm water. Continue to hand mix until it becomes dough and then knead slowly for 15 minutes until the mixture becomes soft and smooth. Divide the dough in two equal batches and flatten both, cover each with a towel and keep in a warm place for 45 minutes. The dough is ready to bake when you push in the surface and it springs back. Sprinkle some flour onto a baking tray and put the two batches of raised dough side by side onto the tray. Poke the dough with fork before placing in the oven.

Preheat the oven at 400° F, (204° C) put the baking tray in the middle of the oven and bake for 30-40 minutes.

Wii Love to Compete
Party Mix

1 cup butter
1 tsp garlic salt
1 tsp celery salt
1 box cheerios
1 bag pretzel sticks

1 Tbsp Worcestershire sauce
1 tsp onion salt
6-8 drops Tabasco sauce
1 box Chex cereal (or Crispix)
2 jars mixed nuts

Heat in a 200° F (95° C) oven. Put all cereals, pretzels and nuts in a large baking tray.
Melt and cook all the other stuff in a pan on the stove. Pour melted mixture slowly over the cereals mixture while stirring. Bake in oven for one hour, stirring every 20 minutes. Serve and enjoy!

Sizzlin' Summer Soiree
Colorful Pasta Salad

1/2 cup olive oil
5 Tbsp yellow American mustard
2 tsp garlic powder
1 bag pasta spirals
1 green bell pepper
2 carrots

5 Tbsp red wine vinegar
1 Tbsp dried basil
1/2 tsp salt
1 red bell pepper
1 yellow bell pepper
Any other fresh veggies you choose

While pasta is cooking chop all the veggies. Mix all ingredients, refrigerate. Like most pasta salads, this is even better the next day, so make a day before your soiree. I also like to serve it with plenty of cracked black pepper and feta cheese.

Wild West Hoedown
Taco Soup

2 lbs (907g) lean mince beef or turkey
1 chopped onion
2 cans chopped tomatoes, with juice
1 can red kidney beans, with juice
1 can pinto beans, with juice
1 can black beans, with juice
2 cans shoe peg corn, with juice
1 package dry taco seasoning
1 package dry Ranch dressing mix

Brown meat with chopped onion, pour off any fat and put in slow cooker. Add tomatoes, beans, corn, taco seasoning and Ranch dressing. Bring all to boil, reduce heat and cook on low heat 4-8 hours. Serve with jalapeños, shredded cheddar cheese, sour cream and Tabasco.

Fondue You Want to Come Over for Dinner
Chocolate Fondue

10 oz (300ml) thickened cream
1/4 cup Cointreau liqueur
10.5 oz (300g) dark chocolate, finely chopped
Your choice of fresh fruit (strawberries, banana, raspberries)
8.8 oz (250g) packet marshmallows
8.8 oz (250g) packet pretzels

Heat cream in a saucepan over medium heat until almost boiling and then stir in Cointreau. Place chocolate in a heat proof bowl. Pour hot cream mixture over chocolate. Stir until melted and smooth and pour into a warm bowl. Serve with fruit, marshmallows and pretzels.

Cookie Exchange
Lemon Cookies

1 package lemon (or cherry or chocolate) Supreme cake mix
2 eggs
1 small container of whipped topping (cool whip)
Powdered sugar for coating

Mix all ingredients together and roll into balls then roll in powdered sugar. Bake in 350° F (180° C) oven for 10-12 minutes.

Suggested Song Lists

Miss-Mix-A-Lot

You wouldn't take a shot of tequila without lime and salt (we assume), and you wouldn't have a night of learning to mix good drinks without some of your favorite drinking songs. So here are some of mine - the first one isn't a 'drinking song' per-se, but it seemed appropriate to start you off with Sir Mix-A-Lot!

"Baby Got Back" **Sir Mix-A-Lot**
"Funky Cold Medina" **Tone Loc**
"Brass Monkey" **The Beastie Boys**
"Tipsy" **J-Kwon**
"Raise Your Glass" **P!nk**
"(Cheers) Drink to That" **Rihanna**
"Hippy Hippy Shake" **The Georgia Satellites**
"Tequila" **The Champs**
"Whiskey River" **Willie Nelson**
"Margaritaville" **Jimmy Buffet**
"Gin and Juice" **Snoop Dog** (or the version sung by **The Gourds**)
"One Scotch, One Bourbon, One Beer" **Amos Milburn**
"Family Tradition" **Hank Williams Junior**
"Friends In Low Places" **Garth Brooks**
"All I Wanna Do" **Sheryl Crow**
"All Summer Long" **Kid Rock**
"Red Red Wine" **UB40**

Karaoke Queens

Back in the day, when I travelled regularly to Manhattan, my dear friend Nookie and I would frequent Japa's, the world's-best karaoke bar near the corner of 55th and 8th. Japa's is an unassuming place with a very long bar where you can usually get a seat and they bring you the microphone when it's your turn so you don't have to get up on a stage. Lots of Broadway-hopefuls come to Japa's and they are hard to follow when you can't carry a tune in a bucket, but after a few drinks no one really minds and Nookie and I would belt out a few hits. The following is a set list of my favorite songs to karaoke:

"Naughty Girls" **Samantha Fox**

"Hurt So Good" **John Mellencamp**

"Livin' on a Prayer" **Bon Jovi**

"Like a Virgin" **Madonna**

"Sweet Caroline" **Neil Diamond**

"Suspicious Minds" **Elvis Presley**

"Faith" **George Michael**

"You Never Even Call Me By My Name" **David Allen Coe**

"Hard to Handle" **The Black Crowes**

"Maneater" **Hall and Oates**

"I Will Survive" **Gloria Gaynor**

"Lady Marmalade" **Christina Aguilera, Lil' Kim, Mýa and P!nk**

"All the Small Things" **Blink 182**

"American Girl" **Tom Petty and The Heartbreakers**

"The Weight" **The Band**

"Ants Marching" **Dave Matthews Band**

"To Be With You" **Mr. Big**

Around the World

While the following list doesn't hit all seven continents, it does represent a good selection of countries and their popular songs and artists. The list is skewed to the USA as it is my home country and I happened to live in three states that all have great songs about them. A nod to nostalgia!

- Africa - "African Drums" **African Tribal Orchestra**
- Argentina - "Libertango" **Astor Piazzolla**
- Australia - "Down Under" **Men at Work**
- Brazil - "Mas Que Nada" **Sergio Mendes and Black Eyed Peas**
- Canada - "Home" **Michael Bublé**
- China - "Mo Li Hua" **Orchid 18**
- Cuba - "Gantanamera" **Joseíto Fernández**
- England - "Werewolves of London" **Warren Zevon**
- France - "La Vie En Rose" **Édith Piaf**
- Germany - "99 Luftballons" **Nena**
- India - "Aashiyan" **Shreya Ghoshal and Nikhil Paul George**
- Ireland - "Beautiful Day" **U2**
- Iceland - "It's Oh So Quiet" **Bjork**
- Italy - "Tu mi porti su" **Giorgia**
- Jamaica - "One Love" **Bob Marley**
- Middle East - "Arabic Medley" **Salaam**
- Mexico - "La Bamba" **Richie Valens**
- Russia - "Russian Jigga" **Seryoga**
- Spain - "Bailamos" **Enrique Iglesias**
- Sweden - "Dancing Queen" **ABBA**
- USA - "Sweet Home Alabama" **Lynyrd Skynyrd**
- USA - "Country Roads" **John Denver**
- USA - "Carolina in My Mind" **James Taylor**

Viva Las Vegas

There are lots of songs about 'Sin City', gambling and money, and a few of my faves are listed below. I've also thrown into the mix a few up-beat songs that will keep you pumped up when you're winning!

"Viva Las Vegas" **Elvis Presley**

"Luck be a Lady" **Frank Sinatra**

"Come Fly With Me" **Frank Sinatra**

"Poker Face" **Lady Gaga**

"The Gambler" **Kenny Rogers**

"Little Less Conversation a Little More Action" **Elvis Presley**

"Papa Loves Mambo" **Perry Como**

"(I Can't Get No) Satisfaction" **The Rolling Stones**

"Money" **Pink Floyd**

"That's the Way I Like It" **KC and the Sunshine Band**

"Born To Be Alive" **Patrick Hernandez**

"Yeah!" **Usher featuring Ludacris and Lil' Jon**

"Live Your Life" **T.I. featuring Rihanna**

"Sweetest Girl" **Akon featuring Lil Wayne, Nia and Wyclef Jean**

"Take the Money and Run" **Steve Miller Band**

"Money Honey" **Clyde McPhatter & The Drifters**

Ice Cream Sundays

An old-fashion ice cream parlor would not be complete without an old-fashion jukebox belting out some sweet tunes. For your Ice Cream Sunday make sure you load up your jukebox (iPod, CD or record player if you don't have the real thing) with songs about ice cream, sweets and a few 1950's throwbacks. Here are a few suggestions:

"Ice Cream" **Pixie Chicks**

"Ice Cream Freeze (Let's Chill)" **Hanna Montana**

"I Want Candy" **Bow Wow Wow**

"Tutti-Frutti" **Little Richard**

"Ice Cream" **Wynton Marsalis and Eric Clapton**

"Ice Cream Man" **Van Halen**

"Ice Cream" **Preservation Hall Jazz Band**

"Sugar Sugar" **The Archies**

"Lollipop" **The Chordettes**

"Rock-in Robin" **Bobby Day**

"Coconut" **Harry Nilsson**

"32 Flavors" **Ani DiFranco**

"Ice Cream" **New Young Pony Club**

"Milkshake" **Kelis**

"Pour Some Sugar on Me" **Def Leppard**

Bond Girls

Whether your covert party operation is going to be more Austin Powers than 007, it is essential to score the evening to help set the mood. The following are a few popular songs about spies and secret agents along side a few themes and songs from famous spy movies.

"Soul Bossa Nova" **Quincy Jones and His Orchestra**

"Theme Song from Mission Impossible" **Danny Elfman**

"Secret Agent Man" **Johnny Rivers**

"Independent Women" **Destiny's Child**

"The Pink Panther Theme (Original Version)" **Henry Mancini and His Orchestra**

"Live and Let Die" **Paul McCartney**

"The James Bond Theme" **John Barry**

"Espionage" **Green Day**

"Blues for Mother's" **Henry Mancini**

"Bullitt Main Title (Movie Version)" **Lalo Schifrin**

"Am I Sexy?" **Lords of Acid**

"Main Title - Goldfinger" **Shirley Bassey**

"From Russia with Love" **Matt Munro**

"Dr Evil" **They Might Be Giants**

"It's the Hard Knock Life (Ghetto Anthem - Dr Evil Remix)" **Dr. Evil**

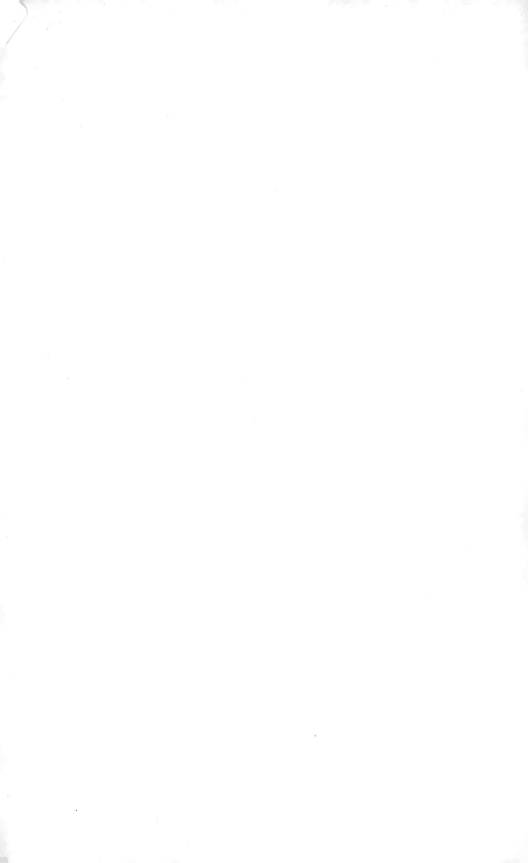

Made in the USA
Charleston, SC
25 October 2013